Hope

MW00436423

Ultimately What You Need
From Your Doctor

5/4/23

Dear Ruth,
I look forward to
Walking this journy to better
health along with you!

In Health,

Dr.

Hope and Healing

Ultimately What You Need From Your Doctor

By Jean Golden-Tevald, DO

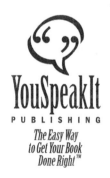

YouSpeakIt
PUBLISHING
The Easy Way
to Get Your Book
Done Right™

www.YouSpeakItPublishing.com

ISBN: 978-1-945446-25-2

Dedication

To my husband, Bill, my beloved partner in this adventure called Life.

And to my children, who are a grand part of that adventure: Elizabeth, Galina, Andrew, Nadia, Brian, Vitaliy, and Irina.

Acknowledgments

To my team: the staff members over the years who have loved our patients and have made a practice culture of love, respect, and caring. You have given our patients hope and healing. Thank you for supporting me to be the best doctor I can be.

Thank you to my business mentors at FPC who helped us see that there is a way to deliver top-notch medical services that help make these services sustainable.

Thanks to Keith and Maura Leon, and all the staff at YouSpeakIt Book Program, for helping me bring these thoughts to the printed page.

Because the apple does not fall far from the tree, thanks to my parents, who always taught me: if to be right is to be different, by all means, be different.

Contents

Introduction

Have you ever wondered how to find a really good doctor?

Maybe you've tried to find one to help you with a troublesome health problem. You may not have had to do this yet, or you may have had this experience with a friend or a loved one. That's what this book is about: finding the best doctor.

I wrote this book because after more than twenty-five years in family practice, I learned many things from the patients I encountered. I grew and changed from my experience as a physician. I realized that many patients had come from unsatisfactory relationships with their doctors.

I continually strive to do a better job to meet my patients' needs.

I have decided to share what I think many patients are looking for, and what I have learned in my approach to:

- Diagnosis
- Treatment
- Problem-solving
- Relationship-building

I want you to have a better understanding of what is possible.

As you go through the book and read each chapter, ask yourself:

- Does the material resonate with me?

- Is this expression a need that I or my loved one has?

- Does the approach to the problem sound like the way I would like to go about handling it?

Put yourself in the different scenarios. I hope you will gain a peek into what it might be like for us to sit together in my consultation room and explore your situation. I want you to feel encouraged and empowered to tell your story. Your story is what guides the therapeutic relationship, and the journey to full, optimal health. That's what you deserve.

I hope that you will be encouraged to strive for optimal health and to pursue a relationship with a doctor who will help you feel the best that you can.

CHAPTER ONE

Reignite Hope

MANY PATIENTS HAVE LOST HOPE

Suzie has come to my office with a stack of paperwork from past consultations and labs. She's filled out her health questionnaire, but she's not feeling confident because she's been to many doctors before and told them her story. She hasn't felt that she's made any progress. This is not an uncommon kind of presentation.

Patients from many similar situations start by telling me that they don't know where to start. I give them time to tell their story, and tell them to start from *now*. I ask how they are feeling now. Then, we go back and look at where they've been.

Sometimes giving a patient that space allows her to feel confident that she is going to be heard this time.

That feeling of hopelessness—*Maybe I can't find an answer*—is common, and it's unfortunate.

When we try to discover and fix the underlying cause, the issue may be infertility, your hormones may be out of whack, or you need a good family doctor to help find diagnoses and provide support.

What are some of the scenarios we deal with in our practice?

Couples Who Struggle With Infertility

There are two common problems that arise when working with couples who struggle with infertility. If you and your partner are working to solve this problem, you may have been through the typical fertility workup, which usually means first seeing your local gynecologist. You are told to try for a year and come back if you haven't conceived.

A year later, you may undergo several basic tests and a couple rounds of the fertility drug Clomid, and then get referred to a fertility clinic. When you go to a clinic, you expect to get an in-depth evaluation and answers to why you have not been able to conceive.

When you eventually come to me, you may tell me there was no in-depth evaluation. You may have received a series of treatments that ended with several rounds of unsuccessful in vitro fertilization (IVF).

Or, you may seek additional consultation because you do not want IVF for moral reasons, or to interfere with the natural conception process. So you come seeking a fertility program, like NaPro TECHNOLOGY, in which we seek to find the underlying cause of your problem.

No matter which problem you have, your NaPro TECHNOLOGY evaluation includes:

- Having your story heard
- Education in how to track fertility
- Developing a treatment plan

When you see how much the biomarkers of your own body reveal to us, the problems we have identified will bring you hope. Your treatment plan will feel like a logical next step.

Negotiating Perimenopause and Menopause

Perimenopause can be a difficult time. It begins when your cycles start to change and continues until a full year after your last period. In order to appreciate that process and the difficulties, you first need to know what normal function should be. Some women enter perimenopause with a dysfunctional system. But even if everything was working fine, as you get into your forties, there will be subtle changes in your menstrual cycle.

Long before you start to have changes in the length or interval of your cycles, there will be a decrease in the amount of progesterone that your body makes after ovulation. During that phase, we can support your cycle in a way that cooperates and works very well *with* your cycle.

Then you enter into a period that I call *no man's land*, when your cycle becomes very irregular. You start to skip periods. There might be several months between cycles. During that phase, your hormone levels are quite unpredictable. We do the best we can to balance what is usually estrogen dominance by using natural progesterone.

Natural progesterone helps to balance hormones, which prevents heavy bleeding and feeling out of control. As you transition to full menopause—when you haven't had any periods for a full year—then it's much easier to look at your individual situation.

Is there a need for additional bioidentical hormones?

We assess that on an individual basis.

Being a Detective in Chronic Illness

I enjoy working with patients who have chronic illnesses and are having a hard time discovering the underlying cause. This analysis requires looking at the whole person.

We don't look just at the results of your:

- Blood labs
- Digestive function
- Hormone function
- Sex hormone levels
- Adrenal hormone function
- Insulin levels
- Other stress hormone levels

We ask:

What's going on emotionally?

How is your social history affecting your life?

We look at all of your systems together, not just your:

- Digestive system
- Cardiac system
- Musculoskeletal system
- Respiratory system

This is one of the benefits of being a generalist physician. We can send you to a specialist, if that's needed, to further evaluate specific problem areas.

Often patients come with a stack of consultations from their specialists, including:

- A rheumatologist
- A cardiologist
- A pulmonologist

Specialists look at your health through their own lens. This is similar to the story about the blind men who each feel a part of an elephant. They try to describe what an elephant is, but all come up with different answers because each is only feeling one part of the animal.

That frustration of only being looked at in one way is part of why the real answer to a problem hasn't been found. This frustration can lead to a feeling of hopelessness.

You may think: *Nobody knows what's going on with me.*

Each specialist has a different opinion.

ANSWERS CAN BE FOUND BY LOOKING OUTSIDE THE BOX

You can usually find the answer if you are willing to look outside the box. If the answers were simple in the more complicated troubles you may have — infertility, difficult transitions through change of life, or complicated chronic disease — you would have found them a long time ago. The standard medical approach includes diagnostic testing and then medication to address the symptoms. However, it is necessary to go back upstream and see what the contributors are to the dysfunction of your body.

We need to look at basic processes, such as your:

- Energy system
- Nervous system — because it's all connected
- Nutritional intake
- Emotional state

Mainstream medicine that uses diagnostic testing and medication to deal with symptoms isn't very good at balancing these other areas. However, these systems are key to understanding and improving the function of your whole body's health system.

There Are Many Sources of Medical Knowledge

There are many different systems of health knowledge, such as:

- Western
- Chiropractic
- Herbal
- Ayurvedic — a traditional Indian whole-body healing system

Sometimes, the challenge is that the specialists in these different areas of health only look at you, the patient, through the lens of their methodology.

Again, it is critical to find a physician who is willing to look at and appreciate which of these other complementary therapies might be appropriate for you. We can take the best tools in a big toolbox and use them to help your situation. If all you have is a hammer, everything looks like a nail. Physicians don't always want to look at the complementary therapies, and the complementary therapists don't want to look at mainstream medicine. However, using the whole toolbox can be very helpful.

I'm an osteopathic physician. A strong part of osteopathic training is a holistic view of your body. I think this view contributes to an open-mindedness about complementary therapies.

We have tools in our toolbox with which we view your:

- Musculoskeletal system
- Interaction of the autonomic nervous system
- Visceral systems

Learning to Trust Your Own Body's Signs, Such as Fertility Appreciation

In our culture, most women have been indoctrinated to distrust their body's signs.

This distrust occurs in spite of how much we say, "Listen to your body. Be in tune with your body."

For some reason, fertility problems cause a great amount of fear.

Mainstream culture tells you to be sure to take hormones and drugs to suppress your fertility system, or to make your fertility system do what you want it to do, because it's really not to be trusted.

When you learn to observe your body's signs, the one thing that you come back to tell me is that you can't believe you can know this much about your body and how it's functioning, just from these simple observations on a day-to-day basis!

It's been great to see patients have that reaction, whether they're twenty, thirty, or forty-five years old. Women in their forties say they wish they knew this ten or twenty years ago.

That brings a good feeling for me, knowing you see the value of learning at this stage of your life.

Don't Expect Everyone to Agree With You or Support You

Going outside the box to find answers to your problems may make people around you feel threatened or uncomfortable. Your choices might be different from their own.

Don't be too surprised if people who are close to you — your family or your friends — give you a hard time about examining alternatives. They're not living with your situation. Don't let them discourage you from seeking the help that you need.

Most patients are excited to hear that we're going to be looking at problems in a different way, either because they haven't heard of the alternatives before, or they haven't been encouraged enough in the past.

IF YOU WANT DIFFERENT RESULTS, YOU HAVE TO DO SOMETHING DIFFERENT

In the areas of sexuality and fertility, there are many individuals or couples who are unhappy with their intimate relationships.

They may:

- Be trying unsuccessfully to have a baby

- Need to postpone pregnancies during their childbearing years

- Be in a relationship, but seek a lifetime marriage partner

Our culture gives us this message: You must control your body and its fertility.

We are also told that there are no consequences to the decisions we make. You should be able to completely separate what you want from what you get.

The truth is if you want something different—a healthier, more intimate relationship—how you handle your sexuality and fertility may need to be done in a different way.

It's Hard to Step Away From What Everyone Else Has Done

Birth control, the most widely used form of family planning, suppresses the natural functions of our body. It is also used to manipulate the body to super-ovulate, or to control the fertilization process. What we're proposing in NaPro TECHNOLOGY is a very different way of going about either family planning—to avoid or achieve pregnancy without any problems—or to help a couple discover their underlying problems and allow the woman's body to function naturally. It's a different road from what most people have been exposed to.

The Creighton Model FeritilityCare System

The Creighton Model FertilityCare system is a method of fertility appreciation and evaluation. The beauty of it, beyond providing the woman with the knowledge of what the different signs of her cycle mean, is that it opens up a channel of communication between a husband and wife. The couple learns to appreciate their ability to bring a new person into the world, and to carry this heavy responsibility. Knowing potentially fertile times can help the couple enter into this decision-making in a way that is pretty awesome.

They realize: *If we come together now, we might create a new person.*

If it's important for them *not* to bring a new person into the world at this time, it allows the couple to make the decision to postpone a possible pregnancy. The decision-making process allows intimate communication, which is what builds a strong partnership. The Creighton Model is a vehicle that allows that sharing and mutual decision-making to occur.

The Creighton Model is the charting of fertility signs:

- Days of bleeding
- Presence or absence of cervical mucus

NaPro TECHNOLOGY is the medical application of what we see on the Creighton chart to drive medical decision-making, diagnoses and treatments. Some people use the Creighton Model only to track their signs. They don't have any problems; they don't need NaPro TECHNOLOGY. If you have a medical problem or concern, you bring your chart to us, and we provide evaluation and treatment.

NaPro TECHNOLOGY

In modern women's health practices, most of the problems that women present—whether irregular cycles, PMS, or irregular bleeding—are given a solution of a one-size-fits-all, suppressive treatment. Nine times out of ten, not even an underlying diagnosis is sought, let alone *made*. The beauty of NaPro TECHNOLOGY is that in addressing a woman's reproductive problems, we seek to find and fix the underlying problem to restore normal function.

The woman comes to understand why something is not working well, and why she's not feeling well. Of course, fixing the problem helps her feel better, both physically and psychologically.

Patients are ultimately excited and empowered when they realize they have alternatives. These options are greater than what has been offered to them in mainstream medicine.

CHAPTER TWO

It's All About Relationships

RELATIONSHIPS TAKE TIME

In today's culture, everything seems to be about efficiency and getting the job done quickly. Relationships
don't work that way.

Beyond the Seven-Minute Visit

If you've been to the doctor lately, you might have
noticed that appointments are getting shorter and
shorter. Many publicly traded HMOs during the
1990s, for example, reduced doctor-patient visits to
seven minutes.[1] Patients have shared with me how
unsatisfactory this is. That hurried feeling of trying to
relate all the concerns that you have to a doctor you
may not know well does not seem to be an effective
way to solve your problems.

It is very unsatisfactory to try to understand a patient's
concerns in seven minutes. There are only two situations
when I've been in that scenario, because I don't do it

---

[1] nytimes.com/2006/03/22/opinion/the-doctor-will-see-you-for-
exactly-seven-minutes.html

in my own practice. However, I have worked in urgent care, and I have done *locum tenens*, which means stepping into another practice to cover for a physician who is out. I have had both of these experiences in the last two years. It was amazing how I was expected to see and treat a person in that short a period of time.

This time constraint places a lot of pressure on both the doctor and the patient. You may try to blurt out your story, and the doctor may try to cut to the chase and get at what they think is important. It's pretty easy to go down the wrong path, because of the way you have told your story in the first few minutes. Your attempt to condense your story to provide it as quickly as possible may not have provided key information.

Giving You Time to Tell Your Story

One piece of sage advice that I remember from my mentors when I was in medical school and becoming a doctor is:

If you listen carefully enough, the patient will tell you the diagnosis.

After more than twenty-five years in practice, I can say that this is almost always true.

The patient doesn't always know what the diagnosis is, or what parts of their story are the most important.

Asking open-ended questions and allowing enough *time* for a patient to relate their concerns can often lead to the diagnosis through this talking process.

The story — and how you tell it — is a very important piece of arriving at a diagnosis. You can't rush it, or you're going to miss important parts of the narrative. Sometimes a person who has been to multiple doctors for their current problem has not obtained a satisfactory resolution. When they're given the chance to tell their history and their concerns in an unhurried way, they'll often remember things that they never had a chance to tell before that are relevant.

Creativity in the Treatment Plan

One of the best tools in developing a relationship with a physician is having enough time and space for your story to unfold. As we start to put together a treatment plan, the same thing may happen to me. I will share what my thoughts and recommendations are and have enough time to explain them. As I get to know you, I may receive additional ideas about how to help improve this plan for you.

Your feedback can help modify the plan in a way that is particularly relevant and acceptable to you. It's a back-and-forth process between you and me. Your treatment plan will not be a one-size-fits-all proposition.

The time that this takes doesn't have to be inordinate. Sometimes, a very good relationship can be forged in one day or one encounter. Or it may take many encounters. The key element is it needs to be enough for you.

BUILDING MUTUAL TRUST

Just like any important relationship, there has to be a level of trust to have an open, honest relationship. In the patient-physician relationship, it has to be built both ways for it to be most effective.

When you come to me with your concerns, I think you realize that you need to be honest about what you share with me. Sometimes you might not realize that it's also important to share not just what is happening or what has happened, but how that has impacted your life.

I want you to tell me:

- What you're scared about
- What you're worried about
- What you've already tried before
- What you are currently trying to do about the problem

You may decide to omit something because you're embarrassed about it or you think it won't be accepted as reasonable, but that can get in the way of me being able to help you.

It's also important for me, as your physician, to be honest and authentic with you. I listen to your story in a nonjudgmental way. Even in unorthodox approaches or unreasonable fears, there may be a kernel of truth. It helps me to understand your perspective.

Trust Builds Over Time

Trust in relationships develops over time. As we each are honest and authentic with one another, it helps us feel more comfortable in the relationship. You don't have to worry about what I'm going to say, or if I'm going to follow through with what I've said I'm going to do. The same thing is true for you.

You may feel uncomfortable with something I recommend to you:

- A test
- A change in your lifestyle
- A medication

In which case, I would like for you to say to me:

- This is not going so well.
- I'm concerned about this.
- I don't think I can do this.
- I don't want to do this.

When this communication is open and free, it builds trust. I believe that if you say you're going to do something, you will. You trust that if I say I'm going to do something—follow up with you or look something up for you—I will. These are the kinds of things that increase the trust in our relationship.

One of the beautiful things about the trust built up over time in the doctor-patient relationship is that if there is a crisis—a major medical concern—it is so reassuring to have a relationship with a physician you know. You can reach out to them in that time of crisis. Even if they're not your attending physician, you value their insight, because of the way your doctor has gotten to know you over time.

Taking Care to Preserve Trust

I try to be especially careful that if I tell you I'm going to do something for you, I follow through and do it.

You can trust me if I say I will:

- Call you in two days
- Get you the results of this test back to you when they come in
- Talk to your daughter
- Be present
- Be there when I say I'm going to be there

These actions are critical for preserving trust. Sometimes, a patient will break trust, but I think it's more devastating to the relationship if the physician doesn't follow through on what they said they were going to do.

THE SATISFACTION OF DEVELOPING A THERA-PEUTIC RELATIONSHIP

Efficiency and speed sometimes seem to hold the highest value in our modern world.

Is a trusting relationship still important?

I feel it *is* important, because it's not just about a warm, fuzzy relationship, but also about a therapeutic relationship. A therapeutic relationship is one in which complete healing can take place.

A Therapeutic Relationship Helps Both of Us to Be Better People

A therapeutic relationship can open your eyes to the importance of having a doctor walk along your journey of healing with you. In today's information age, *Doctor Google* is called upon many, many times, but you usually don't get a very therapeutic relationship with Doctor Google.

You need to have a good doctor who sees all of your worries.

This is true from my side, too. By helping you in your journey to feel better, I become a better doctor. Developing a deeper understanding of how my patients respond to the challenges in their lives and by treating you as unique helps me appreciate your individuality. It's not a cookie-cutter method.

A Therapeutic Relationship Matures Over Time

As we get to know each other and understand our responses to the challenges of life that come up, we learn the nuances and responses of the other person. This helps our relationship mature and grow to deeper levels. In some relationships we *click* or understand each other much more readily than in others.

But even when it takes longer to get in sync, the maturation and deepening process can still occur. It's very satisfying when it seems as if we start in far-apart places but come to understand and appreciate each other.

In this next section, I will discuss patients who were harder to click with.

The Story of Brenda

I think of one patient in particular. Her name is Brenda. She is a scientist and a very driven person. She and her husband came to me with infertility. Brenda *wanted everything yesterday.* Her job had been causing her tremendous stress for a number of years. I tried to communicate with her that in order to let her body heal and bring her to a state of health that would increase her chances for pregnancy, she was going to need to slow down.

We ended up doing some additional testing of her adrenals to prove to her how dysfunctional they were. We worked together over a period of about two years. She saw a hypnotherapist and really concentrated on her control issues and other problems.

This is unusual for what we would normally do with an infertility client, but to see her grow and change over those two years was tremendous. During that time, Brenda and her partner did not conceive. However, she became much healthier and happier, and her relationship with her husband was much improved. We both felt very satisfied that we had really grown in our relationship together, and I was able to help her with her health.

The Story of Agnes

The second patient who comes to mind in this challenging development of a relationship is a patient whose name is Agnes. Agnes and her husband are from Poland.

The easiest way to describe Agnes would be in this statement: "We are going to do it my way."

She had a way of being demanding to all our staff — front office, educational, clinical, and even myself. We were all put off by her demanding ways of interacting with the office. But over time, we developed a relationship. She was also an infertility client.

I was able to see Agnes's emptiness inside and how her demanding exterior was a defense against being hurt internally. We have been working together for about two years, and she and her partner have not yet conceived. There are multiple medical problems that are the cause.

However, Agnes has softened, become in touch with herself, and has come to understand her own health and why some of her issues may be interfering with the couple's ability to conceive. This result has brought a level of satisfaction to the relationship that in the beginning I never thought could occur.

It Never Gets Old

There is a certain satisfaction that occurs when a relationship doesn't take off strongly right away, but instead develops over time. You and I might have very different approaches or worldviews of how things should be done, but we work to achieve some mutual understanding. That understanding is very satisfying.

In relationships that are easier — when we have a similar approach in the beginning and that *click* happens right after the first encounter — both of us feel like we've gotten our therapeutic relationship off to a good start. But it doesn't just stay on cruise control. It has to be constantly nurtured. That process never gets old, because people — both you as the patient and I as the physician — are not static or stationary. We continue to learn or experience events that change our perspectives.

The beauty of a good, trusting, therapeutic relationship is that every time we have an encounter together, there's always that possibility to share what is new or to question an approach that we've taken before. That's what keeps the relationship from getting stale. Continuing to be open and honest with each other helps to keep our relationship fresh and helps it continue to be positive and therapeutic.

One of the neat and satisfying events of my practice is that sometimes I'll have an appointment with a patient whom I haven't seen for many years; maybe even five or ten years. The patient may have moved away or other events have occurred in their life, and they haven't been to the practice in a long time. But something comes up, and they want to come back to our relationship because of the trust and the relationship that was built there in the past.

They may ask "Do you think I should do this?"

Or they tell me, "I went to a specialist, and this is what they recommend. What do you think?"

It always amazes me when people see a top specialist in a field that I'm not an expert in, but they want my opinion because we have a relationship of physician-patient trust.

CHAPTER THREE

A Woman's Health Needs a Special Kind of Understanding

A WOMAN USUALLY HAS EXCELLENT INTU-ITION WHEN SOMETHING IS *NOT RIGHT*

The topic of intuition is so important because it is usually what initiates the encounter with the doctor. Your intuition often includes problems not seen on the outside.

For instance, you may experience:

- A cut on your leg
- A change in the color of your skin
- Something that's externally visible

It is more common that it is a problem you experience internally. Your sense that something is wrong and needs attention is so critical to bringing the problem to the forefront so it can be evaluated and treated.

Issues With Fertility and Hormonal Health

Although you usually know that something is *not right*, you may not know what the problem is. Because as women, our individual experience is just that — our *own* experience. Things like the normality of our menstrual flow, the normal feelings that we have as we go through a cycle — whether you want to call that PMS or shifting of how we feel through the month — we have only our own experiences as a comparison.

So even though you talk to your friends and your family members, your description of heavy flow or menstrual pain is in the context of your own experience. Hormone health is the *least* specific of the intuitions that women have about their health. Fertility is certainly an obvious example. If a couple wants to conceive and is initially unsuccessful, a sense of *something is not right* comes up easily.

One of the challenges that I see in so many women is that when they *do* identify that they're having trouble with their fertility or their hormonal health and reach out to a physician for help, many times the physician does not pay enough attention to diagnose the underlying problem. Rather, solutions are suggested that are just Band-Aids to cover up the symptoms. Likewise, in assistive reproductive technologies, they just go around the problem and try to help a couple get pregnant. This lack of attention to the *why* is very frustrating to the women in my practice.

Issues With Mental Health — Depression and Anxiety

Anxiety and depression are subjects that come up frequently in my discussions with female patients.

They realize that their mental health affects the other people in the family, including their:

- Spouse
- Children
- Extended family
- Siblings
- Parents

That old saying, "If Mama ain't happy, ain't nobody happy," rings true.

I think maybe that's why women are more open than men in discussing challenges with depression and anxiety. I'm not sure if we experience a higher frequency of anxiety and depression, but women seem to be more open to admitting that it's interfering with their lives. Women are open to exploring how to feel better, so that they can function better within the context of their family and community.

Even if you are more willing to discuss these problems, there is still an element of stigma for a lot of women.

You may discuss it, but still be reluctant to accept the diagnosis. Helping you see how your mental health can be tied to your hormonal health or other physical problems that are exacerbating anxiety or depression can also help to normalize your experience a little bit.

At least you may see: *It's not all in my head; there is something not right going on in my body. We need to figure out what that is and fix it.*

Nine times out of ten, this perception will also help you feel better.

Issues With Chronic Fatigue and Pain

I often see patients with chronic fatigue and pain, especially in mid-life — women in their forties and fifties — although it can affect women in earlier and later years as well. These are major contributors to anxiety and depression.

Again, I think these symptoms cause the most distress because they interfere with a woman's ability to do what she perceives as the important work in her life, whether that is:

- Work outside the home
- Work raising her family
- Volunteer work in the community

Chronic fatigue and pain are challenges that are invisible to those of us on the outside. I am amazed at how women with this kind of condition can put on a good face and get through the key things that they need to do. However, they really suffer for it later, when they're at home and not in the spotlight.

That invisibility makes it hard for the other people in your life to realize that you're struggling. Realizing that this level of fatigue or pain is not normal and can be helped is what can drive you to seek medical help.

That same intuition that is key in bringing you to seek medical attention also works for other family members. If you worry about your child or have brought your husband to see me, I listen very carefully to that concern. The intuition that works well for you also works very well for your family members.

I think that this intuition is an important *early warning system* for the family. You can call it *mother's intuition,* but a woman's intuition serves a very important purpose in the health of a family. Your doctor should accept that you have this intuition. They may need to have the hardcore evidence before looking into a symptom and point out that you don't have a fever, for instance. You need to say there are other symptoms, even if they are hard to describe.

Sometimes patients tell me about an experience that they had when the doctor was very dismissive of their intuition. That attitude usually drove them to see another physician.

SHE OFTEN UNDERESTIMATES HER OWN NEEDS

I think this intuition is important for all the people who touch your life, whether it's professionals working with you, your spouse, or your children. We sometimes expect people are very straightforward and if they say yes it means yes. If they say no it means no, and if they say, "I don't really need that," it means, "I don't really need that."

In many years of working with women who are trying to feel better or get healthy, I've learned they often put others' needs in front of their own; sometimes, to their great detriment.

It's Okay to Take Care of Yourself

I think women are wired to be caregivers.

We care for our:

- Children
- Spouses

- Aging parents
- Brothers and sisters when they get into trouble
- Animals when the children won't take care of them

There are only so many hours in the day. Often, our own needs get relegated to the bottom of the list. I'm surprised at the level of guilt some women feel about taking care of their own needs. I think most are just afraid of being perceived as being selfish or uncaring. Sometimes not taking care of yourself can be dramatic, and far out of proportion to what most people would think is *normal*.

For instance, you might sleep only two hours a night—not because a sick child needed you during the night. That would be a normal thing to do. It might be because the house needs to be cleaned or you are performing another daily living task that does not require caring for a family member.

It's dramatic the actions that we can put off, which many of us would just think of as basic self-care.

My message to you is the same as my message to many of the women I work with:

It's okay to take care of yourself.

Not only do you deserve it as a human being, but also it's necessary if you're going to maintain or regain your health.

It's Okay to Invest Time and Money in Your Own Health

In order to take care of ourselves, it usually takes some time, if not money.

We all only have so much time and so much disposable income. We need to prioritize what needs attention and care — first, second, and third. If one of the children needs shoes for baseball — a specific kind of shoe that costs eighty dollars — that task might go to the top of the list, as opposed to purchasing a supplement or a medication that might be necessary for the woman's health. I am amazed by this.

A patient might tell me that a treatment is not covered by insurance. That will usually prompt a conversation which begins with this question:

What is insurance about?

Insurance is to help protect you against the big expenses. It doesn't mean that there will not be any out-of-pocket expense. Thirty dollars a month isn't that much to spend for progesterone, for instance.

Progesterone:

- Helps your hormonal state
- Helps your mental health
- Helps your physical health
- Normalizes your periods

I am amazed at how often women need encouragement from me, as their doctor, to say, "You're worth it. Your health needs to be a priority for you and for your family."

When put in that context, I hope you will see it clearly. But sometimes encouraging you has to be very explicit, far more important than writing you a prescription.

Take Care of Yourself to Take Care of Everybody Else

I think there has been more attention given to this issue—caring for the caregiver—in the last fifteen or twenty years. It's probably because we now have a bigger *sandwich generation*: women between forty and sixty-five who are caring for aging parents who are living longer and their own children. This generation has also expanded as couples delay child-bearing. Everything happens at once: the teen years of your kids, children still in grade school, and elderly parents. Menopause can occur in the middle of it all, just to make life more challenging.

You might be a caregiver of aging parents. They might have dementia or other significant needs. You might be trying to care for them in their home. Even if they're living in assisted living or in a somewhat supervised environment, you are still taking them to doctor visits and worry about their health and welfare. You take care of some of the financial details, and a full-time job on top of it all makes things a little more fun. It's really easy to push the limits of your own endurance.

When I get the sense that part of a woman's issues is that she's just really overwhelmed, I'll ask her to tell me what usually happens on a Monday.

I'll take her through the day:

When does she get up?

When does she eat?

What happens next?

What happens on a Friday or Saturday?

As she's telling the story of what her day is like, it becomes obvious to her that this pace is kind of crazy. This method has been helpful to get women to see that their actions are really beyond what would be expected.

If you are one of these women and want to continue to do these things, you are going to have to take care of your own health needs, or it's just not going to work.

This is usually the easiest tool to give women. Having them actually *do* it—invest time and money in themselves, and actually do things to care of themselves—is a little bit more challenging. Helping them see that they need to take care of the caregiver, and receive permission to care for themselves, is an important part of my job as their physician.

Sometimes a woman will bring her spouse either to the initial consultation or a subsequent visit. I really like it when her partner comes along, for a couple of reasons. One, I can see some of the dynamics of their relationship, and that helps me to understand the woman as my patient.

The second reason is that one of two things tends to happen. One is that the spouse is *not* aware of my patient's level of needs. Unfortunately, those are usually the partners who don't come.

But the partners who do come are the ones who see that she needs support and are there to be another voice to say, "See, honey? The doctor is right. It's okay for you to do x, y, and z."

Your spouse can actually be my best ally in helping you see what needs to be done and not feel so guilty about taking the time to take care of yourself.

It's interesting to note, especially in the NaPro work with fertility and hormone health, the couples who end up coming to our practice. We don't just cover up the problem with birth control pills or go around the problem with IVF. Our type of approach brings us a lot of couples in which the spouse is truly concerned about the wife's health.

The partner wants to make sure that my patient is not given medications or treatments that might be harmful to her, even though there might be other outcomes that they want. When the spouse is so protective of her health, it's sweet to see her cherished and cared for.

I think that kind of caring is a byproduct of our approach to women's health problems.

SHE OFTEN NEEDS HER DOCTOR TO VALIDATE HER NEEDS

A lot of patients who come to me have already been to other doctors. I'm a family doctor, so I have a generalist training. I also have more specific training and experience, especially in gynecology and hormonal problems. I might not be the most obvious selection when someone is going through a list of specialists and doctors.

Many people do self-refer to specialists, so if they think they have a thyroid problem they go to an endocrinologist. If they think that they have a hormone problem, they see a gynecologist. If they were having a chronic pain problem, they probably would go to an orthopedist. Those doctors are not always the best entry points for those problems.

Perhaps you have already been to at least one other practitioner, and perhaps more than that. Those experiences keep you searching for help with your problem because it has been minimized. You may have been told that you don't really have a problem.

Let's look at an example of a thyroid problem. One blood test, the TSH, or Thyroid Stimulating Hormone, comes back within the normal reference range. You are told that your blood test is normal. There's nothing wrong with your thyroid. End of story.

It certainly can be much more subtle and complex than that.

One of two things can happen. Your sense of intuition is still very strong, and you realize that something's still wrong. This doctor is not giving you the right answer, and you keep looking for an answer.

Or, you accept the diagnosis that there is no problem.

You suffer silently, thinking: *This is just the way it has to be.*

Those who come to us looking for better answers really appreciate the validation, "Yes, something is wrong."

We might not know what it is yet, but we will keep looking, and we'll figure it out. It might not be what you think the problem is, but if you don't feel well, something is not right.

It's Not All in Your Head

As part of our NaPro TECHNOLOGY workup, we first teach you to chart your fertility cycle: the way to observe external signs of your body that reflect what's going on biochemically in the hormones of your body. You chart that on a day-by-day basis. Then we do a targeted hormone profile, which consists of blood tests every two days from the time of ovulation through the two weeks afterwards. We look at what the levels of hormones — estradiol and progesterone — are, and they should follow a specific pattern.

There are certain patterns associated with many of the hormone problems, such as:

- Endometriosis
- Infertility
- PMS
- Heavy bleeding
- Changes of perimenopause

When we put your results on a graph of what should be normal, and you can see clearly where it's abnormal, the impact is amazing. Of course, we explain what the results are and what they mean. It is powerfully validating to have that piece of paper that shows clearly what the problem is and where the problem is, and then discuss what we can do to normalize it.

This is not an easy thing to do. When you do these blood tests, you need to know where you are in your ovulation cycle and you need to know what *normals* are. These are not the *normal* levels that are on blood tests from Lab Corp or Quest. Those are ranges that include the whole cycle. You do need to have the norm to compare it to, and that comes out of research from the Pope Paul VI Institute in Omaha, Nebraska. It is very rewarding to be able to show you the results on paper. You will also track your symptoms as you go through the cycle of the hormone profile.

You can see the shift of your own symptoms.

You may experience:

- Insomnia
- Breast tenderness
- Irritability
- Headache

But you can look at the blood test results and see exactly where it shifts.

It's tremendously validating to help you realize it is not all in your head. Something is happening in your body that is causing you to feel differently.

You Have Something Special to Offer to Your World

I really believe that women have many different kinds of genius, if you want to call it that. Each woman needs time and space to figure out what it is that they have to offer their world.

Sometimes it's in:

- A professional capacity
- An artistic capacity
- An emotional capacity — how she relates to people in her family, her community, or in her workplace

There are different kinds of leadership. In recent years, our culture makes a greater acknowledgment of the value in the many contributions that women make to our world. It's not just in the home, or just in the workplace, but it can also change through a woman's lifetime, in how she shares her gifts with her community.

Part of my job is helping you see that. Sometimes I do this through the process of evaluating your physical problems, and I can be just one more person who can validate your gifts. I can see how your unique talents in leadership are something special that you share with your Girl Scout Troop, for example.

Taking care of your health and helping you feel better so that you can make that contribution is important to me. Sometimes the validation is not just about your illness or your dysfunction, but it's also about your role in your community.

I'll Help You Get Better—I'm Not Giving Up on You

That sense that *we're in this together* is really important, especially in some of the situations that are not so easy to correct.

Two of these situations come to mind. The first is chronic fatigue.

Chronic fatigue can emerge from different things:

- Injury
- A viral infection
- Adrenal fatigue from long-term stress
- Infertility, where a roller coaster of hope and despair happened repeatedly

The second is infertility. After an initial consultation or workup, most patients have high hopes. Sometimes, things do get better very quickly, or couples conceive or have a successful pregnancy, but not always. I let them know that, of course, my goal is to help guide them and figure out what's wrong and to fix those problems as much as possible.

One of the things that I usually tell my patients is that as we go forward, I want them to know everything that I know. I give them a copy of all their labs.

When we do an ultrasound, I show you exactly what I'm looking at and explain what it means. As my patient, you will understand how NaPro works on a day-by-day basis. You will see the signs and symptoms that are unfolding, and understand what the results of your different tests mean. I will teach you this since it's our journey together.

You may become discouraged. Sometimes discouragement comes sooner; sometimes it comes later. Sometimes it comes after a procedure like endometriosis surgery. If conception doesn't happen after that, discouragement can come roaring in. I will let you know that my biggest concern is helping you and walking with you.

I will be there to give you a pep talk, lift you up, and encourage you when you're feeling down. One of the things about medicine, especially the more complex situations like chronic fatigue, chronic pain, and infertility, is that doctors sometimes get discouraged, too, or we run out of tools in our toolbox. If we're going to do the job correctly and stand by you, sometimes that means reaching out and helping you find other resources to bring to bear on your case.

It's not telling you that I am dismissing you and sending you to Dr. Smith, but rather suggesting another opinion from Dr. Smith that we will talk about and see if that would be reasonable to consider.

I let you know that just because things aren't going the way we hoped they would, I'm not going to give up on you.

CHAPTER FOUR

It's a Journey Together, and I Want to Help You Help Yourself

LOOKING UPSTREAM FOR THE CAUSES OR TRIGGERS OF DISEASE OR DISCOMFORT

It is usually symptoms that bring you to the doctor's office, but it's important for you to know that just focusing on what you're feeling now very rarely gives you the answer. As we go forward, looking upstream, or at what came before the symptoms, often gives us the clue to a solution.

A Functional Medicine Approach

What is a *functional medicine* approach?

Most people would expect, when you come to the doctor's office with some symptom, that you would be offered a solution or a treatment that will make that symptom go away. That's what mainstream Western medicine primarily does. It is helpful in crisis situations, but not so much for chronic disease. *Functional medicine*, which is a newer term—you might not have heard it before—focuses on how your body functions, and helping it to function well. That's where the term *functional medicine* comes from. The diagnosis does not focus on just the symptoms that you are experiencing.

How do we do this? Basically, I start by listening to your story and finding out why you're here.

After going over what you're experiencing right now, the next questions are:

- What happened before that?
- When did you last feel well?
- When did you notice things turning for the worse?

We will keep going back, and back, and back in the story, either until we find the time when you really did feel well, or sometimes *way* back, even to childhood, and it turns out that some of the triggers or things that set your body into the motion of not working well happened quite a long time ago.

Those triggers include:

- Events
- Injuries

- Accidents
- Severe illness

The cause might be all kinds of things, but digging deep into the story for those times when your health changed is going to be important in finding the solution and helping you get well again. This is the functional medicine approach.

We also look for *mediators*, or the things that keep a dysfunction going.

Why doesn't your body just get better on its own, which it is usually primed to do?

There may be things in your environment, or in your diet, or in your psycho-social environment that are keeping you from getting well, and we're going to explore those, too.

Predisposing Genetic Factors

As doctors achieved a better understanding of underlying genetic factors, we thought that this was going to be a big part of the answer to help cure disease and improve people's health. But it turns out it doesn't exactly work that way. There are certain predisposing factors. If you look back in your family history — your parents, your grandparents, and your extended family — there certain types of diseases present.

You might have a family history of:

- Heart disease
- Cancer
- Addictions
- Mental illness

Your genetic dispositions are not your destiny. We're starting to understanding that there is much more. There are what we call *epigenetic factors*. These are chemical tags that indicate what, where, and when genes should be activated. However, the choices that you make in your lifestyle can actually overcome a lot of these predisposing genetic factors. It is important to understand where your genetic vulnerabilities are, but they are not your fate, and that can be good news.

How Do Things Tie Together? Not Just Treating Symptoms

Now that we're looking at your whole story — what your family history might be or your genetic vulnerabilities — we consider more.

We look at what has happened:

- In your life
- In your prenatal life
- In your infancy
- In your childhood as you entered adulthood

We're looking for what are triggers—causes that have set things in motion the wrong way—and what are mediators—causes that are keeping things going in the wrong way. We can focus on these specific areas of dysfunction and work to repair them, in order to remove the obstacles that allow your body to heal itself.

Our bodies have an innate ability to repair and heal themselves. Sometimes the treatment is getting out of your own way, and removing the things that keep the dysfunction going. The problem could be in your gut and how you digest things, or in your mind and how you think about things. Tying together all of these pieces sets us on the journey to healing that is empowering.

We have many medicines that will mask a symptom. Sometimes it is necessary to use medicines and get a symptom under control while we work upstream and fix some of the ongoing factors that are contributing to disease. But to just treat the symptom without looking further leaves you dependent on symptom management medications for life, and that's not a very satisfying solution.

THE CHOICES YOU MAKE ARE POWERFUL

When we're looking upstream for the triggers of what's ailing you, we often discover that it's not just the trigger that is the only cause. Certainly the mediating factors, or the things that keep things going in a less-than-ideal way, are the choices that we make.

Every day, we choose:

- What we eat
- How we move
- How we deal with challenges in our lives

We'll look more specifically at each, and see how the choices we make affect our health every day.

You Are What You Eat

You'd have to be living under a rock to not know that nutrition and what you eat is important for your health. But I am amazed how much misinformation and conflicting information is out there. Most people are pretty confused about what constitutes a healthy diet.

A big part of health education is a clarification of how our bodies take the food that we eat and process it so that we can:

- Repair tissues
- Grow
- Have plenty of energy

What are pitfalls we face when choosing what we eat?

You might be surprised that it's quite a bit different than what the food pyramid has promoted for many years.

Move It or Lose It

I think one of the biggest changes in our modern lifestyle, other than the addition of processed foods in our diets, is a decrease in personal activity level.

If we think back to a more agricultural society, when you got up early and worked in the field or outdoors, you:

- Carried things
- Ran away from things
- Had to push things around

I'm sure our ancestors never thought about exercise.

Today, we:

- Drive our cars to the gym
- Work out at the gym
- Drive our cars home
- Sit in front of our computers before we go to bed

If we feel like we're exercising three days of the week when we go to the gym, that's nowhere close to the level of activity that human beings once had in the normal course of their day. If we want to consider activity, and the level that is important to maintain our health, we need to think about the big picture of how we move our bodies, not just think about *exercise*.

Dealing With Challenging People In Your Life

Probably the third biggest area that affects our health on a daily basis, besides nutrition and activity, is stress.

There are many forms of stress:

- Physical
- Chemical
- Emotional

What causes the most emotional stress for people? For you?

If it's dealing with the other people in your life, it is productive to go through the process of looking at the people in your life, and how you think about them.

Sometimes, part of my job as your physician is to help you look at those relationships and identify the patterns of behavior that have developed. The patterns become habitual, and we don't consider that perhaps there's a better way to deal with these other people.

These patterns are an important part of managing stress on a day-to-day basis. It's one of the choices that you make. You can choose to be angry or not, you can choose to work out a problem or not, and you can choose to forgive someone or not. This awareness is going to be an important part of your health choices.

The Story of Suzi

Suzi came to me because she was developing multiple medical problems:

- Diabetes
- High blood pressure
- Depression
- Overweight

Suzi is a professional architect. As we got to know each other, I realized that Suzi was taking care of everybody else, but she wasn't taking care of herself. She also wasn't getting support for her own needs from the other people in her life, particularly her husband.

Her problems came to a head one day when she was physically exhausted. Her blood sugar was out of control, her hemoglobin A1C was over eight, and she was clearly diabetic. I had to discuss this with her and tell her that she now had diabetes. She *had* to take care of herself.

Suzi wasn't seeing how the relationships with other people in her life — her husband who was not supportive and her son who had become disabled and angry —

were negatively affecting her health. She was taking on the brunt of these negative relationships. We continue to this day to work on these problems. Helping Suzi see how her other relationships were having a negative effect on her life really helped her take control of her health and start to move it in the right direction.

The Story of Janet

Janet, an infertility patient, and her husband were a little older in their reproductive life. She was forty-five by the time they came to us, and unfortunately they had had a tragedy in their life. They had a daughter who was five years old and had heart surgery. In the post-operative period, she developed an illness and died in a very unexpected way. This had happened three years before I met them.

The couple desperately wanted to have another child, but Janet was still actively grieving the loss of their daughter and was so angry at the medical system and a messy lawsuit that she was totally dominated by these negative feelings. As we got to know each other, she came to understand that because of her age, her chances of another pregnancy were slim.

I realized that one of the most important things I could do for her and her partner was to help them heal from the loss of their daughter. We talked about it many times. The couple understood that even if Janet were to conceive again, no other child could replace the daughter they had lost. I encouraged Janet to also go to therapy, which she did to a certain extent.

I hope she will continue to engage in therapy. But sometimes our job as physicians is not just to deal with the patient's medical condition, but to help see how their emotions are affecting their physical health. I hope Janet will continue to grow on the road of healing from the grief of the loss of their daughter.

LOOKING FORWARD TO A LIFE WITHOUT DE-PENDENCY ON DOCTORS AND DRUGS

As you grow older, you may expect that you will accumulate a list of medications. If you hang around doctors and hospitals long enough, you will certainly feel that way. It doesn't have to be that way. One of my very favorite things is taking care of people in their seventies, eighties, and nineties who don't have a medication list.

You may have one or two medications you need to take. It's not because you've chosen not to deal with issues, but your body is actually functioning quite well. You may have some supplements, and that certainly is one of the things that can help your body function better and reduce the dependency on drugs and medication.

Let's look at how you can look forward to that kind of life.

Your Doctor Can Do Only 5 Percent of What Needs to Be Done

It's important to understand the role of medicine in long-term health and vitality.

What is the role of your physician or your healthcare advisors?

My job is really 5 percent of what needs to be done. Sometimes it's a very important 5 percent, because it's the 5 percent that helps you identify what the problem is, and develop a treatment plan or a course of action to take. So I don't mean to downplay the importance of that 5 percent. It would be foolish to not seek out that 5 percent of the solution if you are having a problem, but it is not the whole solution.

As we work together on a treatment plan or a course of action, you must monitor yourself. If something is not going right or your day-to-day activities don't seem to be getting the results that you expect or are causing more discomfort, it's time to come back to me and ask for more guidance. We're going to talk about independence and personal responsibility, but part of that personal responsibility is to know when to ask for help with the 5 percent.

You Have to Do the Other 95 Percent

Clearly, if I can only do 5 percent, somebody else is responsible for the 95 percent.

Guess what?

That's you.

It can be a little bit overwhelming, especially if you always thought medical care meant your doctor would solve your problem for you.

Occasionally it does, but with more chronic disease issues, there's a lot more to it than that.

The 95 percent is what you choose to do every day:

What you eat

How you move

How you deal with stress

My job—besides pointing you in the right direction for what to do, especially in those three areas — is to provide education. Doctor Google is usually not your friend or best advisor when it comes to sorting out how to apply lifestyle changes to your own life. I look forward to that education helping you be more effective in the choices that you make every day.

On the one hand, it can feel scary to have that much responsibility. But the flip side is that it's empowering to know that you do have control over many things about your health, and that you don't have to just be a victim of destiny, disease, or the medical industrial complex.

We Can Do It Together

The best part about embarking on this journey toward a life without dependency on drugs and doctors is that we can do it together. You don't have to shun medical care or be reluctant to seek out advice because of what might be offered to you. I have known people who have ignored very serious symptoms of disease due to the fear they'd be told that they'd have to take certain medicines for the rest of their life, or that it would demand a level of dependency that they did not want.

But I look at it in a very different way as your doctor, education is the major part of my response to you. Certainly, it's exploration and diagnosis, but the next biggest part is educating you about how to care for yourself with the condition that you have.

There's no need to fear, and it's an active, vibrant process of education and communication. I hope that it will be an empowering journey for you, and not something to be feared.

You don't have to be perfect. Do the best you can. We sometimes regroup or readjust the plan, but it's a dynamic process that is meant to be engaged in.

Let me say it again. You don't have to be perfect.

Some medical problems seem like life sentences:

- Diabetes
- Heart disease
- High blood pressure

Just because you got onto that ride doesn't mean you have to stay on it forever. You can often get off by dealing with the upstream causes. What drives the health care system — or *sick care system*, if you want to call it that — is money. Money drives many things in life, so if Big Pharma gets you on a long-term medicine, what's the motivation to get you off it? Pharmaceutical companies certainly profit from the medication.

And profits come from anything that feeds the medical system, such as:

- Doctor visits
- Testing
- Hospitalization

Changes in insurance, such as the Affordable Care Act, have affected patients' fears and thoughts about their medical care.

You would think that their biggest fear would be: *I need insurance, heaven forbid I need surgery or hospitalization.*

Actually the biggest reason that people are keeping their insurance is medication. The cost of medication is surprising. The prices of medications have skyrocketed even for meds that used to be cheap like thyroid medicine or simple antibiotics — not the fancy ones, the simple ones. The price of thyroid medication, which is one of the ones you may need to be on forever, used to cost the patient about ten dollars a month. Now the patient cost for generic thyroid medication is about seventy dollars per month.

That's just not right.

In many cases there aren't many choices other than the easier lifestyle answer of: *I don't need that medication.*

In the past, the cost of generic medication used to be much less than a brand-name med. That discount still helps a lot. However, it is ridiculous for a patient to have to pay seven hundred dollars a month or more for three generic medications. These are the costs is what people are facing.

Here is the choice: *Do I buy my three diabetes medicines at seven hundred dollars per month, or do I buy organic food and join a gym? That's five hundred dollars a month.*

The medical system certainly says that you need your medication, and sometimes you do.

I'm not saying that medication is never appropriate, but investing in lifestyle education and change can save you money and heartache down the road.

CHAPTER FIVE

Healing Is Always Possible, Even If A Cure Is Not

WHAT HEALING IS

If we want to understand the doctor-patient relationship or encounter, we need to understand the goal. Healing is the ultimate goal of a healer.

We need to clarify what, exactly, is that? What exactly is healing?

Definition — to Ease or Relieve Suffering

The word *patient* in its original Latin means *one who suffers.*

The person who comes to a doctor for help is someone who is suffering either physically or emotionally, and at first, we're not clear where that suffering is coming from. How we ease or relieve that suffering is what healing is. That's not necessarily the same as *curing* a disease. To *cure* – also originating from Latin, *cura*, or *care* — means using something such as a drug or medical treatment that stops a disease and makes someone healthy again.

To cure would be to remove disease, or to make the disease process go away or be resolved.

Healing is to relieve the suffering that the person has, and that doesn't necessarily have to come from a cure. If a cure happens, it also doesn't necessarily have to come from healing.

Considering our overall view of well-being and care, expectations are important.

What is the expectation of the physician?

If it's only to cure, and not necessarily to take the patient to full healing, the patient is not going to be fully satisfied. The same presents for the patient: if they are expecting only a cure, a full cure may not be possible. Helping them come to an understanding that a full cure might not be possible, but to continue to address their suffering and handle that appropriately, is also the job of the physician. This sometimes helps guide the patient in the process of what is the appropriate and expected outcome, and to communicate that effectively.

Understanding the Underlying Condition Leads to Healing

If we are trying to help relieve suffering that a patient is experiencing, we need to understand the underlying conditions. We want to understand the underlying physical and emotional dysfunctions and challenges. We want to understand some of the spiritual issues that a patient may be experiencing.

The Story of Sarah and Chris

I'll use the example of Sarah and Chris. These patients were a couple in their early thirties who had been married for several years, and had been unsuccessful in having children. Two doctors they had visited previously saw that Sarah had regular cycles. Some basic testing did not show any clear reason for her infertility. This would be a case of unexplained infertility.

In the course of their evaluation and subsequent treatment, quite a few things came to light. One was an underlying physical problem called *endometriosis*, which needed hormonal support and surgery.

It turns out that her husband also had some moderate male factor issues that needed surgical intervention and medical support.

But the couple also had spiritual issues to address. As a Catholic couple, there were certain procedures that are often done in infertility — not to fix the underlying problem, but to try to help a couple achieve pregnancy — that were not acceptable to them. It was important, as part of their healing process, to work with medical professionals who respected that view.

They eventually did go on to have a healthy pregnancy — and subsequent pregnancies after the underlying conditions were revealed and fixed — but it took three-and-a-half years for them to get to the point of that first pregnancy. Walking the emotional journey with them was a critical part of their treatment and their feeling of healing. It wasn't just the pregnancy that led to their healing.

Healing Relationships Can Be Vital — The Story of Ethel

The flip side is a situation where it becomes clear that a cure is not going to occur. An example from my experience is a story about a patient I will call Ethel. She had advanced colon cancer, and she fought valiantly. She went through oncology treatments that involved surgery and chemotherapy, despite her advanced age of ninety-two years old. It was important for her to fight hard. It came to the point where it was clear that the treatments were no longer slowing down the growth of the cancer.

In meeting with her and her family, it became clear that she had a number of things that were important to her. One was to be able to be with her family and her extended family, and for her to be as cognitively intact as possible. She didn't want to have her level of consciousness impaired, but she also had physical issues that caused her great pain.

As we negotiated her final care, pain management was really important. The trusting relationship that we had built up over the several years prior made it possible for her believe that I would do my best to help her meet both of her goals: to manage her pain and be as present as possible with her family. Ethel also wanted to stay in her home for her final days.

We were able to achieve these goals. It gave great comfort to Ethel, as well as her family and extended family, to know that the relationship we had built prior to her illness—but then also strengthened through her terminal illness—would help her to have a positive experience until the end.

HEALING OFTEN REQUIRES GUIDANCE

Sometimes it's not clear to the patient what it is that they are seeking. Ultimately, they are looking for healing from the healer, but sometimes they think that the cure is the only route to that healing. My job, as a physician, is to be more deliberate or explicit in helping them see that there may be more than one way to achieve healing in their life and in their circumstances.

Physician as Healer—Your Physician Should Be There to Guide You

A physician's role as healer is what separates a physician from a technician, for example.

A technician can:

- Find a problem
- Diagnose a problem
- Find an appropriate treatment
- Apply that treatment

But a physician's role is really to guide a patient through the process of diagnosis, and to choose the right treatment. Medicine is not as black and white as people think it is. In fact, it's very grey. There may be multiple ways to approach a treatment plan, even for a known, specific diagnosis. The physician's role is to help the patient identify what is important for them, and how each treatment plan might help or hinder that. This is a dynamic process that may change as symptoms and circumstances do.

It certainly is not in any way a purely technical process. If the role of the physician is reduced to being a technician, it is a disservice to both the doctor and the patient. There are some amazing procedures that modern medicine has developed, but they must always be administered in the context of the individual patient's situation.

Opening Up and Being Vulnerable in Your Pain Makes Healing Possible

In the beginning, we talked about the physician who needs to guide the patient through the process of choosing what interventions are most acceptable and appropriate.

In order for me to do that, I need you, the patient, to be open and vulnerable. Helping you heal is a very intimate interaction. We must both see beneath the surface needs. For instance, consider a person who has a tumor from breast cancer. There is a level, on the surface, that makes it clear that the tumor is there. It needs to be identified and treated in some way. But it's also really important to know more about the patient's story.

In order for me to help you heal, I need to know your story, including your:

- Fears
- Aspirations
- Physical needs
- Emotional needs
- Spiritual needs

This knowledge is essential to help you reach a place of healing. Maybe it's a cure and a solution, or it may just be a healing without a complete cure, as in a remission. In order for me as a physician to do my best job, I need you to be open about your needs, fears, hopes, and dreams.

Your story helps me do the best job that I can for you.

A Therapeutic Team Is Sometimes Necessary

By spending the time to identify what your multiple and diverse needs are, I often can't fully provide the help to meet all of those needs. That's the beauty of having a therapeutic team.

A therapeutic team might include:

- Surgeon
- Oncologist
- Physical therapist
- Stress management or mindfulness coach

- Psychologist
- Massage therapist
- Acupuncturist

All of these members of the therapeutic team work together to help you achieve a state of healing. Even within our office, our therapeutic team involves our medical assistants, nutritionists, and our office staff to create a healing environment.

We want this environment to be a place where you can feel at home and share your needs openly with us. I love being able to be part of that team, and many times I orchestrate or am a *captain* of the team, overseeing the organization of patient cases. No one person is more important than the other, but it does take some organization. We need to help you use the services of the members of the team in a coordinated way. Our environment always has you as the center of that team, so that it is patient-driven.

THE PEACE THAT COMES WITH ACCEPTANCE

Many patients faced with illness or suffering go through what are known as the *Five Stages of Loss*, identified by Elisabeth Kübler-Ross.

These stages are:

- Denial
- Anger
- Bargaining
- Depression
- Acceptance

These are the well-known stages a person passes through when learning to live with the loss of a loved one, but they also apply to the circumstances of any patient with unresolved suffering.

In the final stage, a patient comes to an acceptance: *This is how my suffering is going to be relieved.*

When acceptance settles into the heart and mind, it can bring a level of peace that is therapeutic, but also unexpected. This level of peace may lead to changing the patient's perception of solutions that may have been previously unacceptable.

Forgiveness as a Catalyst for Healing

One of the things that comes up in my work with a patient is that there is often anger or a grudge, and it needs forgiveness. The resentment might be toward someone else, perhaps a previous physician or medical professional the patient worked with. The outcome may not have gone well, or the way the patient expected.

The patient may need to forgive someone else in their family who has hurt them in some way or whose actions continue to cause hurt:

- A parent
- A sibling
- A spouse
- A child

And sometimes, the patient needs to forgive themselves for the choices they've made in the past. However, what's done is done, and it can't be undone. Working through that process—helping the patient see what needs to be forgiven, and walking them through doing that forgiving—can remove huge obstacles toward healing: emotional, spiritual, and physical.

It's a step not to be made light of or ignored.

Acceptance Frees You to Live Each Day Fully

Especially when your acceptance is less than you hoped for, you may realize that the underlying cause is never going to completely go away. It might even impede your ability to reach a goal that you had originally identified as what you wanted: fertility, for example.

If a certain condition is likely to prevent you from ever being pregnant—for example, a disease that necessitated a hysterectomy, a pretty obvious one in which the cure for infertility will never be achieved — there still is room for healing the loss of biological fertility.

Healing may include:

- Adoption
- Childlessness, but serving other people in other ways
- Making a marriage stronger through other types of love and service

Accepting that a certain road is closed allows you to live each day without using up so much energy trying to chase something that is not feasible.

Another example that is not as extreme would be where the door is not closed — we'll use the same example of infertility — but where the disease processes are pretty severe, or the age of the patient is advanced so that the chances of biological pregnancy are pretty low.

We can work in a way to leave that door open, so we can provide the treatments that support the body and a healthy reproductive system as much as we can. We do those things on a day-to-day basis, but it doesn't have to take a lot of emotional or mental energy.

How I usually express this to the patient is that we'll just do what needs to be done at different parts of their cycle, but they won't have to decide every day whether they should *do* anything. I tell them to just put it on the calendar, put the supplement or the medicine in the pillbox, and get on with life each day.

Live your life, because you're here today. You may be pregnant next month, or you might not, but you're certainly here today, so live each day to the fullest in the state that you're in.

That kind of acceptance of a possible outcome — but not a likely outcome — can sometimes be healing in itself. Not giving up on yourself, but putting the treatment in perspective, can sometimes maintain a balance that frees you up to live each day in the present.

Acceptance Can Help You See a Path That You Didn't See Before

When you stop being consumed by a goal that is neither achievable or likely to be achieved, a door can open, allowing you to see a different path. I have seen that happen frequently in my patients' lives in many different situations where they were so focused on the one thing that wasn't happening, and that finding a cure was not likely to be achieved.

Once they backed off the original goal and asked themselves where the real suffering was coming from in their condition, they were able to consider what we could do to relieve that suffering, even if we couldn't necessarily cure the disease.

At that point, sometimes you can see another avenue for your life, whether it's in your:

- Work
- Relationships
- Opportunities for service

When I see you a year later, it's almost like you have a different life. It's so exciting to see that happen, because healing has taken place even though your disease was not cured. It's sometimes an unexpected benefit of this view of the doctor-patient relationship.

The Story of Emma and Dave

The first story is about a couple, Emma and Dave, who were my patients. They married late in life. Emma was fifty years old at the time of her marriage and came to us hoping to have a baby. She was still having regular cycles, and she learned to chart them.

But we did need to have some pretty honest conversations about the likelihood of having a successful pregnancy at fifty years old. Emma and Dave were very much hoping that God would intervene in their case and were very open to any pregnancy that would occur.

They were such a sweet couple. They very much wanted to be parents and develop that as part of their new life together. About six months into the process, they were presented with an opportunity for adoption. They took a young baby boy into their home, and eight months later, they were completing the adoption of the little boy. I never saw a happier couple. They were beaming from ear-to-ear about the child God had sent them. It is such a beautiful story.

Their resolution was different from what they had initially imagined. They were flexible enough to see this adoption as a solution that some couples may not have embraced.

The Story of Laura and John

Another example is a couple, Laura and John, who also struggled with infertility. Laura had severe endometriosis. She had surgery and multiple interventions, but no successful pregnancies over a period of four or five years. They really did not want to give up. They felt that God had plans for them for parenting.

One day, Laura got a phone call from a cousin who was having tremendous personal problems, and her children were going to be placed in foster care. Laura and her husband stepped up and did a kinship adoption of these two little girls, who at the time were about three and five years old.

The family worked through some challenging situations. Laura and John helped the girls heal, and now their little family of four is very happy. This was such a beautiful solution both for these girls, who needed a safe home, and for Laura and John who really wanted to share their love as parents with children who needed it. They didn't see that path at the beginning, but it opened up for them and they stepped up to the challenge.

Conclusion

Now that we have looked at a number of different aspects of the doctor-patient relationship, I hope that I have been able to open your eyes to the fact that the kind of relationship you might be looking for is possible.

You don't have to be satisfied with a less-than-satisfactory relationship with your physician. I want you to think about what's important to you, and what your goals are — where you want your health to be — and seek out a physician who can journey with you to help you reach those goals. Don't be afraid to ask questions about the doctor's methodology, and what to expect in your initial meeting.

Ask about the physician's approach to problem-solving. Do they see you working together as a team, or is it more directed by what you are expected to do, and what you're told to do?

You might seek a physician trained in NaPro TECHNOLOGY. The other thing you might want to consider is a physician who works in functional medicine. Remember, this type of medicine searches upstream for the cause of disease or discomfort, in more general terms. That's what NaPro TECHNOLOGY does in the arena of women's health.

The gift that I would like you to receive from reading this book is to know that you deserve to have the kind of healthcare that I describe here. I want you to experience the care that helps you achieve optimal health. You deserve more than avoiding disease; you deserve a partner who helps you strive for a much higher level of health and well-being. Be an active participant in seeking out answers and do the things that you need to do on a day-to-day basis. We talked about the 95 percent effort that is your responsibility. There is responsibility on both sides of the relationship, but you don't have to settle for less-than-adequate care.

Next Steps

We invite you to visit our MorningStar Family Health Center website for upcoming events, programs, and a list of resources to guide you on your path to wellness: morningstarfhc.com.

Follow us on Facebook at facebook.com/MorningStarFHC.

Are you ready to take the first steps to embarking on the journey to optimal health?

We host ongoing free seminars on *Stress, Hormones, and Health*. Call our office at (908) 735-9344 to reserve a seat at one of our upcoming talks. You are also invited to make an appointment for an initial consultation.

I look forward to welcoming you to MorningStar Family Health Center!

About the Author

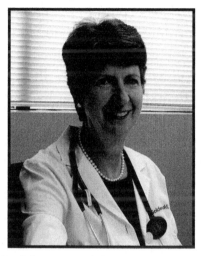

Jean Golden-Tevald, DO, CFCMC, FCP

Dr. Jean Golden-Tevald has been a family physician in rural Hunterdon County, New Jersey, since 1989. After graduating from Barnard College, Columbia University in New York City, she attended the Philadelphia College of Osteopathic Medicine and graduated with her medical degree in 1987.

After a residency in family medicine at Union Hospital in Union, New Jersey, she and her family moved to Hunterdon County to establish a family practice dedicated to relationships and personalized service.

Over the years, Dr. Jean has developed areas of special interest and pursued further specialized training in hormones, functional medicine, women's health, and NaPro TECHNOLOGY.

Finally, the time has come to bring all these threads together in MorningStar's LifeStyle Medicine Program for Optimal Living. She is passionate about helping her patients receive the guidance they need to attain optimum health and change their lives for the better!